Making Love

The complete guidebook to flirting, dating and making love to her

Hienel Farmrich

Legal & Disclaimer

damages, costs, and expenses, including any legal fees potentially resulting from the application of any of the information provided by this book. This disclaimer applies to any loss, damages or injury caused by the use and application, whether directly or indirectly, of any advice or information presented, whether for breach of contract, tort, negligence, personal injury, criminal intent, or under any other cause of action.

You agree to accept all risks of using the information presented inside this book.

You agree that by continuing to read this book, where appropriate and/or necessary, you shall consult a professional (including but not limited to your doctor, attorney, or financial advisor or such other advisor as needed) before using any of the suggested remedies, techniques, or information in this book.

Table of Contents

Overview

Finding a woman of their dreams is what a lot of men want. Unfortunately, many men aren't successful in attracting and loving a woman. This is why I have written this book to help men reach out to women and learn to love them the right way.

The book pays attention to details and will tell its readers even the smallest detail to win over a woman. Women look for a foundation to form a deeper connection and a relationship. It is very difficult to build a relationship with someone who is closed off.

Men who surrender easily have a willingness to step away from the power position that they are raised to feel comfortable being in. They need to learn to embrace the more sensitive things in their lives in order to become the perfect man for their dream woman.

Women are sensitive. In order to attract a woman and win her over, a man has to take certain steps. The readers will come across a lot of information regarding what to do and how to create a good impression on women. A man has to be emotionally stable in order to successfully win over a woman. This means a woman can count on him to be predictable, and reliable.

If a woman feels unequal or silenced in a relationship, then the relationship may not work out. That is why men need to act a certain way to be able to love a woman the way she deserves to be loved. You may be able to successfully reach out to women and develop a graceful image in front of them after reading this book.

There are many dating mistakes a lot of men make. Dating can be hard, but you don't have to make it sound painful. You are going to make a couple of mistakes if you are going to put yourself out there. Sometimes men come off as oblivious, obnoxious, or uninterested even when they're really trying to impress a woman.

The major problem here is they aren't aware of what they are doing wrong. If they were aware of their mistakes, they could actually avoid them. However, dating can be a bit awkward, especially if you've been out of the game for a while. Nobody's blaming you for getting the butterflies.

But talking about how awkward it is will only make the situation worse. You may date a woman for the first time in a number of ways. It may be your first date or a blind date set up by one of your friends. Women fall for a man who makes them feel a certain way. You will know how to have a successful date after reading this book.

Finally, this book tells you what to do when a woman is ready to make love to you, what kind of words to say and what actions to take. It tells the readers that in order to get your woman in a good mood, a man should take her out to a fancy place, and while getting seated pull out the chair for her, in other words, make her feel like a Queen.

Women love these small gestures. Order champagne and pour her a glass. Create a mood and look into her eyes. Give her a smile and make her feel special. After dinner, take her for a drive and hold her hand while driving. Listen to her stories. Women love to be heard. Then both of you are good to go for a memorable night.

The last but not least, at the end of the book, there is a bonus chapter telling you about my most romantic and loveliest experience I have had in love that you can have a look at and apply them into your love life.

This book will create a positive mindset in its readers and will help them understand what a woman actually wants from a man.

Chapter 1: Build a Personality

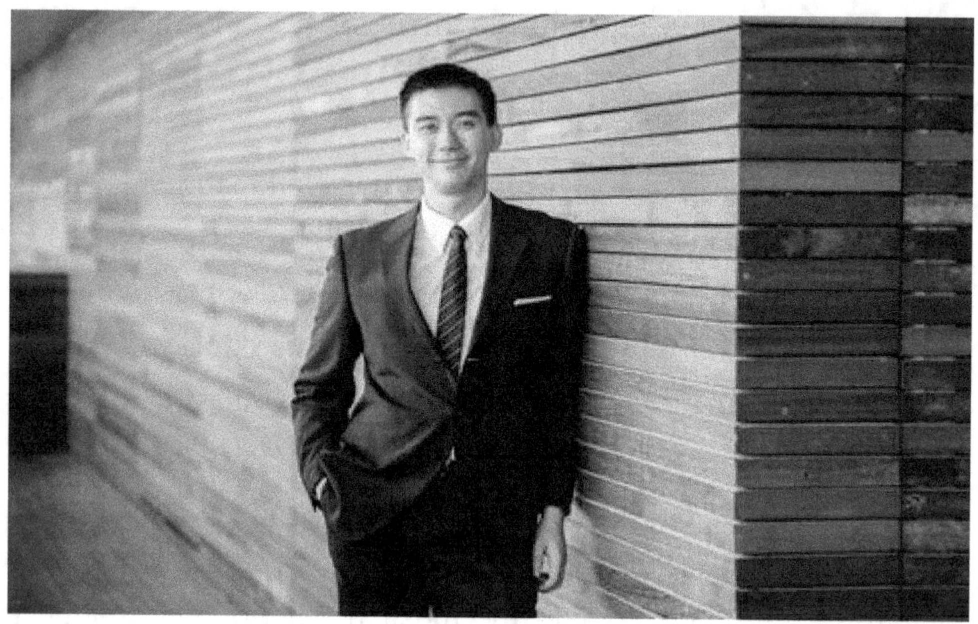

Women pay attention to little details which men do not always give importance to. Attraction, intimacy, seduction, trust, and sex, all of these play an equal part in a relationship. Emotions are the key aspects for a woman whereas men are not very expressive. For a woman, the intention; motivation and authenticity of your feelings matter the most.

In order to win over a woman, you must improve your daily image. You must improve how you feel about yourself and how you express yourself to others. This may sound vague, but to have a good impact on the interactions with women, you have to unmask the attractive and unique person within yourself.

Women choose to be comfortable based on what kind of person they are around. They don't open up in front of men who are just pursuing sex. For men, everything is very straight forward. You may see a beautiful woman and feel aroused. Sometimes you may be pursuing sex, but may not want to have a relationship with a woman. But if you desire a serious relationship with a woman, you may want to feel cared for, admired and respected by her and she will want the same from you.

For women, it's different. They experience sexuality differently than men. This is why it is a lot more complicated for men to understand what really makes a woman get attracted to a man.

In order to develop emotions in a woman's heart you need to first determine the quality of the relationship you have with her. There are a number of ways to attract women. The way you choose will determine the type of woman you will attract.

For instance, if you try to attract women by choosing to be cold, calculating and manipulative, then you will only end up attracting a woman who is cold, calculating and manipulative. Likewise, if you want a woman because you are needy and you idealize them, then you will attract someone who is insecure and needy themselves. The same applies when you pursue a relationship with a woman with a harsh and rude manner. You will only attract a woman who responds to such emotions.

Therefore, always approach women with honesty and authenticity. This way you will attract women who are honest and conscientious. A confident man who has integrity is what women are looking for.

Your whole outlook is noticed by the women around you. The way you talk, dress, smell and the way you treat other people needs to be appropriate in order to attract a good woman and make them feel love for you

Tips on creating a graceful image

Here are a few things you need to be concerned about to make women fall in love with you:

Keep track of what you say

Men are usually very casual and have a habit of using abusive language with their buddies. In a gathering of all males it is not considered to be an eyebrow raising issue. However, women are more sensitive. Using abusive and harsh words in front of them will create a negative image of you for them. They will think you are rude and it will create a distance between you and her.

Women like men who are kind and sober. It doesn't matter if you are a nerd, or affiliated with any kind of sport, or if you are an artist or musician. What matters to them is your words. You require certain communication skills to become a women magnet. You may not know it, but the women around you may be silently noticing how you talk and what words you use.

So, always be a gentleman in front of them. Be nice and kind. Say a big no to abusive words or sentences such as "complete and hand this report to me this afternoon" said in an abusive voice. That combined with a cold bossy face and tone can mark the start of a bad impression of you. And you should absolutely never use any bad words.

However, it can't be faked as that will show immediately. It has to be authentic and honest or no woman is going to be attracted to you for the long term.

Your ways of Dressing

Women pay attention to little details. The way you dress is one of them. You may not pay attention to what you are wearing, but others do. Men often have limited clothes and repeat the same shirts consecutively. This is because men do not find anything wrong with that. However, women are not like this. They will know exactly when you wore that particular shirt the last time.

The point is women notice your style of dress and in order to attract women you need to work on improving it. If you fail to style yourself properly, then you may fail to attract women. Your dress code should be on spot.

Here are some basics to develop a sense of style:

Fitting

Your clothes should fit you properly. Both loose fitting or tight clothes may put off women. If the clothes you buy do not provide the perfect fit, then get them altered. Your clothes should fit your body in a way that they contribute to your personality. Plus the tops you wear should emphasize your physique.

Simple and decent colors

Say a big no to flashy and complex outfits. You may think they would make you look presentable but in reality, they won't. Go for simple and sober dressing with a great style.

Solid colors can never go wrong. For a formal attire, be sure to match the right tie and pants. Never choose loud and showy colors.

Variety in tops

Create a flattering effect with the variety of tops available in the market. You could choose between tees, shirts, vests and sweaters. Choose the right colors and pair them up with an appropriate pair of pants.

Choose the top according to your body type. For example, if you have a bulky body, complex layering would make you look heavier. Choose to wear simple tops that do not make you look larger. Also avoid wearing sweaters and hoodies.
For making your upper body look more appealing you can choose to wear a blazer or a vest instead. If you have a slim body, you can wear extra layering so your physique looks improved.

For a simple and comfortable look, you could choose boat neck tees. For some men, V-necks also work well.

Moreover, if you are wearing a blazer or jacket with a tee-shirt, choose a brighter colored tee. This will have playful, yet exciting look. Above all you want to look well-groomed, and natural, never fake or outlandish.

Comfortable Pants

Jeans, chinos and khakis are the basic choices in pants. Choose the one which is comfortable and you can easily pair it with the tops you have. While choosing a type of pants, make sure you pair it with the right shoes.

Pants are available in many cuts. It can be regular, skinny, loose, slim or relaxed. Each cut is suitable for a certain age group and a certain physique. For example, slim cut jeans are ideal for men below 40 years of age. Be sure the pants you choose fit properly and aren't either too tight or too loose.

Shoes

For some women, shoes play a very important role in declaring a man's personality. They judge men by observing their shoes. For instance, dirty and not properly polished shoes would instantly create a negative impact.

Shoes complete your look, therefore don't just pay attention to the pants and tops. Men often have a habit of wearing sandals or flip flops everywhere. Well, this does not create a very good impression on women.

Different types of shoes work with different types of outfits. Loafers and oxfords are dressier shoes and work well with blazers, whereas boots look more appealing with leather jackets and western style clothing.

Accessories

The right accessories can enhance your overall look. A well-chosen watch will contribute to your style and give you a more mature look. A colorful pocket square would work best with a blazer for a conservative style.

The smell of your body

First off it is vital to shower daily so you begin with a clean body. Women are very sensitive to smell. Pleasant smells will send positive vibes to them, whereas an unpleasant smell would draw them away from you.

Men sometimes forget to pay attention to small aspects of hygiene. One of them is to forget to wear deodorant. Everyone sweats and it is a natural phenomenon which cannot be reversed. But the unpleasant odor can be controlled by showering every day and wearing some deodorant. Wear a good deodorant. Let it be your best friend, especially if your body is smelly.

Your smell could either attract a women or drive them away from you. Use good colognes that last longer and are good from a woman's perspective. There are certain scents that are more appealing for women. These include scents that have Bay Rum, Basil, notes of leather, lime, vanilla, Tonka Bean and Violet Leaf in it.

Women find these scents to be very attractive. For instance, Bay Rum is a traditional scent that will remind a woman of her dad and as many women always try to find a personality like her dad's in every man, this would make them notice you. Whereas a cologne that has basil in it would have a modern fresh note.

Each of these scents have been proven to make an impact on women. Whatever cologne you use doesn't matter if you forget the deodorant, so once again don't forget to wear a deodorant as you would not want to drive the women away due to the bad odor of perspiration.

Gestures

The correct gestures and the right body language are very important while attracting women. If you want to win over a woman you need to appear more masculine and confident. By your gestures and body language you can silently communicate and make her fall for you.

Women like men who are confident. They would prefer talking to a person who believes in himself and knows his abilities. Show them you are confident by your body language. Raise your head with a slight smile, look straight forward, stand firm with your shoulders up and hands out of your pocket. You can gently strut with footsteps on the same line. Make eye contact and keep eye contact when she is talking to you. Don't chase her.

Try to be a good listener. Men who listen to what women say are admired by women the most. Show small gestures like opening the door for them, let them walk ahead of you, offer your jacket if she is cold and hang her bag or jacket up on the door hook gently. In short, be a gentleman.

Overall personality

Women like men who have a great personality. Get her attention by building up a personality. Your dressing sense, smell, communication skills and confidence, everything will contribute to your overall personality.

To build a strong personality you need to work on the following:

Confidence

Confidence is the most important thing a woman looks for in a man. If you lack confidence, then you need to improve your confidence and self-esteem. Overcome your insecurities. In order to overcome your insecurities, you need to accept them and realize there is much more beyond them. Face your defects by accepting and improving them. Once you are more confident women will start noticing you.

General Knowledge

Not everyone is born intelligent. What can put you ahead of others is your knowledge about what is going on around the world. This will help you be a part of any conversation. If you don't know anything then there will be very low chances of speaking up in a conversation between you and your mates. How would you gain the attention of a woman if you are just in the background? Therefore, knowledge is very important.

Leadership

Leaders are what women are looking for. If you have good leadership qualities and are always leading everyone whether it is a project, a sports game or anything else, you will find yourself to be more well-known by the women around you.

Becoming a leader takes ambition and body language. You can lead while interacting with a woman. However, there is a difference between leading and being bossy. Know the line between both. If you become bossy, women would not be attracted to you and will instead be driven away from you.

The way you treat others

Be kind and generous. Treat others around you with respect. Women like men who treat people around them nicely. Harsh and rude behavior will make a women think you are arrogant and she would not want to talk to you. For example, during eating out in a buffet restaurant, the way you ask the chef to put the foods you choose into your dish, and your eye sights will get your girl's attention.

Do not make it wrong that you think the love you give to her is the main thing and all the other small stuff like how you treat others, such as the bossy way you treat a waiter is not important. The fact is you might be able to hide your personality in most of the main parts of love, but you cannot hide it all the time. Some intelligent girls will just focus on little stuff like this to judge how you are really as a person. Therefore, it is ideal to seed small nice habits now to reap a nice personality for your future love.

Not only refrain from being harsh and rude, but also try to be helpful to the people around you. Being empathic will not only help you become a good person, it will also make women want to be with you in a relationship. They will not only like you, but will also respect you for being kind to others.

If you like a certain woman, then be nice to her, be compassionate and show respect and care towards her. Understand her. Be a good listener and listen to her stories as well as asking about her family and friends. This will make her bond with you. For instance, while talking to my girlfriend on the phone I noticed she was always more excited and happier with her cheerful voice and willing to share with me more stories whenever I talked about her family rather than other matters.

Chapter 2: First Meet Her

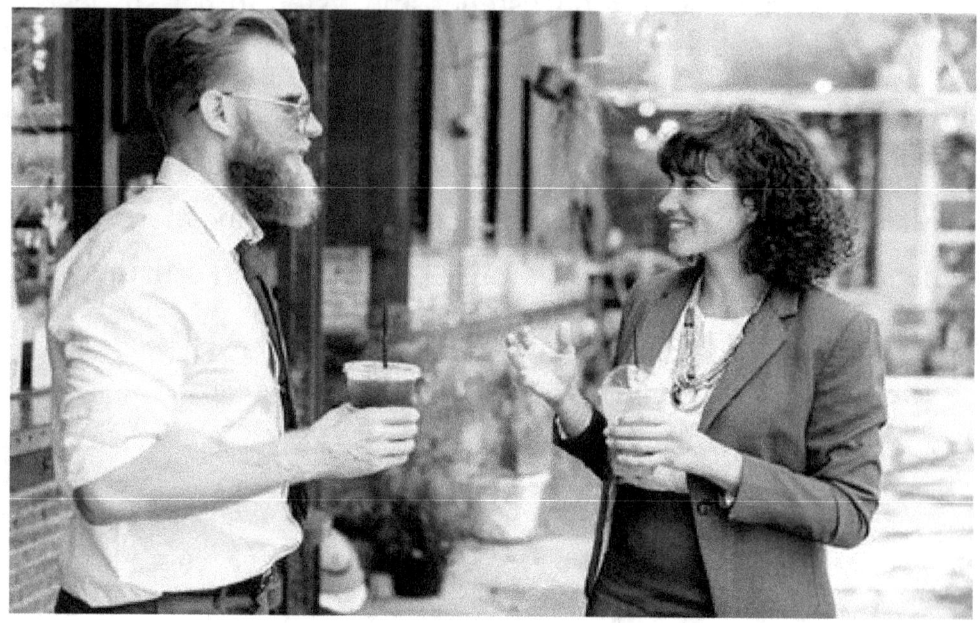

You may find the right woman anywhere. She may be a colleague, a school mate, a neighbor or someone you meet through a friend. If you haven't found the right woman till now, there are various places you could meet someone you have been waiting for. You may meet her on the Internet, at work or by accidents like bumping into her on the street or on a bus or on a train.

The first time you see her; it will be great if she gives you a soft smile with eye contact. This is the signal that she is open towards you. What you can do then is just simply keep smiling gently. If you and her face each other several times later and she looks at you and smiles, then you can consider winking an eye at her.

Meet her on the Internet

You may meet her on the Internet through an online dating site. Women are looking for men on various dating sites just like men are looking for women. To attract woman on these sites you need to make your profile as desirable and engaging as possible. In order to create a fun and engaging profile you must not be lonely, insecure, depressed or sad as these negative emotions will influence your profile characteristics. So pay attention to this when you take your profile picture. And you should not get on the Internet if you are in a bad mood.

Describe the type of girl you want. Be very specific and clear. Sometimes men are not sure and they write on their profile "any girl would be fine." This creates a very bad impact on women. They feel you are needy. So be specific about the type of woman you are looking for. You can simply explain first their appearance like saying you like women with blond hair and blue eyes, then go for the characteristics you desire such as being kind, sympathetic and forgiving.

By doing this, it will filter the women according to the characteristics and whoever reads your profile will get a feeling that you have some standards and know exactly what you want.

The Internet and online dating sites are a fun way to meet new people and make new friends. They allow you to find someone special in a fun way. In some of these sites, there are events such as game nights where you can meet, drink and dance with strangers. These events also let you meet new people who have similar interests. You may find your special someone in one of these events as well.

At your Workplace

Many men find their women at their workplace. They have had a crush on the women since the first time they saw them. You may also have found her at your office. However, you may be looking for ways to attract that woman, but are not getting a chance to do so or are not sure how to go about it.

Finding someone at your work gives you a chance to develop a deeper bond with her as you see her every day. You could impress her in a number of ways. Here are some ways you could create a good impression on a woman you like at work:

Be good at what you do

Whatever your job is, do it with the best efforts. This helps you earn the respect of the woman. Women don't like men who complain, throw tantrums and are careless at work. They like a man who is responsible in his work.

Some men think that being goofy and non-caring would make them look badass and attract women. But this is not the case. Women only like this kind of attitude in their boyfriend or sex buddy. When it comes to a man of their dreams they want them to be efficient at work.

Women like men to be stable and successful. A non-serious attitude at work will make you look like an unsuccessful person. To impress a woman at work, always be productive.

Don't flirt with every woman at work

Women are very observant. You may find a lot of women attractive at work. However, always choose to only get the attention of one woman. If a woman senses that you are a player, she may never want to be with you.

Women hate betrayal. Therefore, they don't want to get affiliated with a player. So, don't try to date a lot of women at work, nor flirt with everyone around.

A woman can find out that you are checking out another woman. Be aware and don't check other women's asses and boobs. In fact, if you really want a woman to respect and love you, don't go straight for checking out her ass or boobs either! It's really not polite, especially in a work environment.

Be nice to her

Women like attention. Make them feel good by making them laugh and smile by telling short stories with a humorous sense or performing magic tricks during break time. These are simple things but they create wonders. Women want a man who makes them feel wanted. You can make them feel great by making them laugh when they are stressed. When she is having a bad day, hear her out. Help her out through her problems.

Make your presence felt, so that when you are not around she misses you and the way you make her feel.

At Bars and night clubs

Bars and clubs are also common in for meeting a woman. Weekends are the best time of the week to visit bars and clubs. It is very likely that you could meet someone on a weekend night at a bar or club.

If you aren't very comfortable in this kind of environment, then you can show up early and get a little hang of the environment. You can chat with the staff or someone who is around to get used to the environment and warm up your social skills.

To find a woman, look for the area with a lot of traffic. It is more likely in a high traffic area that the same woman passes by you frequently. This will make it easier for you to get into a conversation with someone.

Unexpected occasions such as meeting each other on a train, a bus or the street

It is very likely that you may have unexpected small accidents such as bumping into someone on the street or you meet someone on a train or a bus. Just a coincidence can bring you to a woman whom you have always dreamed of.

If such a scenario takes place, all you have to do is start a conversation. It is not necessary or a good idea to start with a pickup line. Just be genuine and honest.

You can just start by saying calmly and warmly, "You look familiar. Have I seen you before? My name is ___________" or "I'm sorry. Are you OK? You look familiar. I may have seen you before?" and don't forget to pick up her fallen belongings while you are asking her. Women look for authenticity and that is what is needed.

What to say first?

Approaching a woman you are interested in can be a little overwhelming. You may want to start a conversation with them, but don't know what to say.

The easiest and the best way to approach her is to find a natural reason. Introduce yourself to her very naturally like, "I am Peter from the opposite table, you dance very well and you look very pretty tonight. Can we have a drink together?"

If she is an office colleague or a classmate or someone sitting next to you on the bus or train, pay attention to what she is doing.

If she is holding a book, try commenting on it to start a conversation.

If she is wearing a stunning outfit, you can come and comment on her accessories. Don't mention things that are near her private parts like necklaces. It shows that you are being sexually interested in her and makes her feel threatened and insecure. Instead, comment on her shoes. The further away from her private parts the better.

All you got to do is to start a conversation by making some small talk with her. From this, you can actually find out if the woman is actually interested or not. It could be anything like asking about the weather, a work project, an event or just the latest news telecast.

Her reaction and the length of her response will give you an idea if she is interested or not.

You can initiate the conversation by saying, "Hey did you see the soccer game last night?". This would lead to an interesting conversation. In case the woman says no she didn't, turn the conversation towards her and ask about if she likes sports or plays any sports.

You can also make a conversation with her if she is sitting right next to you. Say something funny about something or someone and be loud enough that she could hear you out. If she engages in a conversation with you about your comments, then that means she was actually paying attention to you.

The best thing you could go say to her is:

"Hey, I noticed you and I had to come say Hi."

How to behave?

Whenever you see a woman and want to go talk to her always remember that there are certain gestures you could incorporate into yourself to make a good impression on her. This would include:

Eye contact

Eye contact is necessary as it shows confidence and it creates a sense of closeness. When you approach a woman make an instant connection with your eyes. This will show that you are confident and also trigger the production of oxytocin.

Oxytocin is a cuddle hormone. However, a generated eye contact may not create any strong feelings of closeness, but it will develop a sense of trust. But don't use this as an excuse to stare at her, as that is something totally different and it's not something a woman wants at all, and it will make her back away and ignore you.

Approach her from a side angle

Women are at times wary and cautious of men, and may at times be guarding themselves from men. They may get intimidated if you approach them from the front or behind. Always approach a woman from a side angle. This will enable them to see you and prepare for your presence.

Your body language could either make the woman you are approaching feel at ease or either make them feel intimidated. Use body language that shows you are friendly and harmless. Make direct eye contact when you approach her. Move your hands wisely while you talk to her and make them visible to her so that she is assured you are not going to hurt her.

Final things to do to set a deal for the first official date with her.

Once the woman shows interest in your conversations and shows positive expressions such as laughter, smiles and shows open body language, you can ask her out for a date.

If she shows that she is busy, annoyed or closed off, then these are indications she is not interested.

However, if she shows positive signs, then here are some tips on how to ask her out:

Don't fear rejection

Men fear rejection the most. The fear of rejection may make you remain single for the rest of your life. The first step is to overcome this fear and stop overthinking. There are only two possibilities, either she will say yes or either she will say no. If she says yes, then it's great and if she says no, it's not a big deal. Take it easy. Say this to yourself: "If she says no, I am still OK and happy. If she says yes, I will be delighted."

Keep it simple

Don't fall into the trap of beating around the bush when it comes to asking a woman out. Also, don't be as vague as saying, "Do you want to hang out?"

Be specific and straight forward when you are asking a woman out for an official date. This will make them feel that you are serious and are looking for a serious relationship. For example, ask them: "Are you free for coffee this weekend?"

This will make you look mature and confident and there are more chances for her to say yes.

Use your phone to follow up

Build up a communication with her before you take things ahead to the next stage. At this point, phones are the best way to communicate. You can start it all with the help of apps and texting.

Here is a tip, whenever you hear that she is talking with a seemingly sad voice; regardless whether she is unhappy about something or not, ask her why she is unhappy, such as: "Are you being unhappy about something!? My lady, if you have something unhappy, please share it with me, I will help you."

There are two scenarios. The first one is that she doesn't have anything unhappy going on and says: "No, no problem, why do you ask so?" You can reply: "Because I could hear some sadness in your voice. If you have any problems, please share it with me, I can help." Then she confirms that she is fine and then you can tell her if she needs anything, just ask for your help.

The second one is that she has problems making her unhappy and shares them with you. Then you will have a chance to sympathize with her, help her and score a hit in her heart. Whichever the situation is, she will remember your sincerity and admire you because you are sensitive and care about her feelings.

<u>Things to avoid and pay attention to</u>

There are certain things that you must avoid and pay attention to when you first meet a woman. Let's start by talking about a few things that you must avoid:

Do not fake it

Women can sense it if you are genuine or you are faking it. Men often try to fake a smile when they are not actually listening to what the woman is saying or are just hiding their intentions. Do not hesitate to give her a compliment from your true heart like, "oh, today, you look so pretty in that dress" with a cheerful facial express and voice. That can score a hit in her heart. Women like men who are genuine. So never fake anything in front of them.

Eye contact should not be avoided

When it is the first time you have met her, don't avoid eye contact. It is very important to make eye contact. It creates a sense of connection which is necessary for her to develop an interest in you.

When you make eye contact with her, you make her realize you are confident and you appreciate her, respect her and have an understanding towards her.

Do not hide your intention

Be straightforward when approaching her and don't try to hide your intention. She should know that you like her. Don't say it bluntly, but also don't hide it completely. Just try to be natural and authentic as well as friendly and this will help you in getting her attention.

For example, you can say:

"Hi, you look gorgeous, I had to come meet you."

Do not speak in a low voice

Men often speak in a very low voice when approaching a woman. This indicates a lack of confidence to a woman. If you are loud and clear, it will be easier for her to hear you out and simultaneously, it will show her that you are confident. So don't speak in a low voice.

Do not sound boring

No women like to be with a boring man. The biggest mistake you could do is to bore her at the first approach you make towards her. Don't start interviewing her with questions like:

"What do you do?"
"Where do you live?"

Such questions will make you sound interrogative and she would not be interested in dating you again.

Avoid discussion on politics or religion

There are certainly exceptions a woman has when she meets a man for the first time. Whatever she expects, it is not politics she wants to talk about. Men usually make this blunder of talking about politics with them, which turns off a woman and she may get distant from you. Politics is interesting, but it's also exhausting. Even when you both are on the same side of a politically charged issue, bringing it up would remove that feeling of impulsive excitement that comes with a really well-planned date. Save it for a more appropriate setting.

You should also avoid talking about religion, as that's a personal issue that most people feel strongly about and you don't want to offend a woman you are trying to impress.

To create a good impression on a woman, you must pay attention to the following:

Get into the right mindset

Before you approach a woman, you need to get into the right mindset. Don't make yourself sound needy and insecure. For example, saying, "Do you want to have dinner with me?" in an unconfident and influential voice. Women can sense that you are needy and insecure when you are approaching them. You are here to conquer her so make it precise and confident. You can practice the way how you talk to her couple of times before approaching her.

Notice her body language

When you approach a woman, notice her body language. Her body language will tell you a lot of things. If she is smiling and sometimes looks at you with her smile on her face, this is a good sign she is happy and ready to talk to you. If she looks unhappy and cold, you should stand back and wait for another time. You may find out if she wants to be approached. She may not be in a good mood and if you start flirting with her she may get annoyed and snap at you.

Be genuine and honest

Honesty and genuineness are very important. Women don't like men who fake it at all. They want someone who they can trust and rely on. If they sense you are a player, they will never be comfortable with you.

Show respect

The biggest problem women have from men revolves around respect. If a woman feels you do not respect her or other women, there is a very rare chance she will fall for you. Try not to make mistakes like being late or forgetting the date, missing her birthday or any other important things she has told you. And remember to be gallant. Women like men who show respect towards them and don't try to dominate them.

Small details count

Small details matter a lot. The way she is sitting, what she is talking about and what she is wearing; everything matters. Pay attention to little details as they will all contribute towards winning her over.

Be the first one to take initiative

When you notice a woman, try to get her attention. Make the first move fast as the longer you wait to approach her, the less she would react naturally. This will result in making her overthink about the whole scenario, which could then intimidate or annoy her.

Make eye contact

Eye contact will tell a woman that you are interested in her. It also generates a love at first sight. This is helpful in creating an attraction. Eye contact creates a feeling of love and connection.

Maintain a confident polite posture

Men often make the mistake of approaching a woman with a slumped over posture, arms crossed, and eyes facing towards the floor. This creates a very bad image of you. No matter how good a conversation you maintain with her, this kind of body posturing will speak of low self-confidence and bossiness.

Instead, stand straight, pull your shoulders back, keep your head up, and send a message to her that you are a man who is worthy of other people's attention and affection.

Groom yourself

There is nothing better than a well-groomed man. Women are very particular about how presentable a man looks. They judge harshly based on appearance. It doesn't matter if you are well mannered, intellectual, and funny. If you are not well groomed, then there is very rare chance for you.

Chapter 3: Your First date

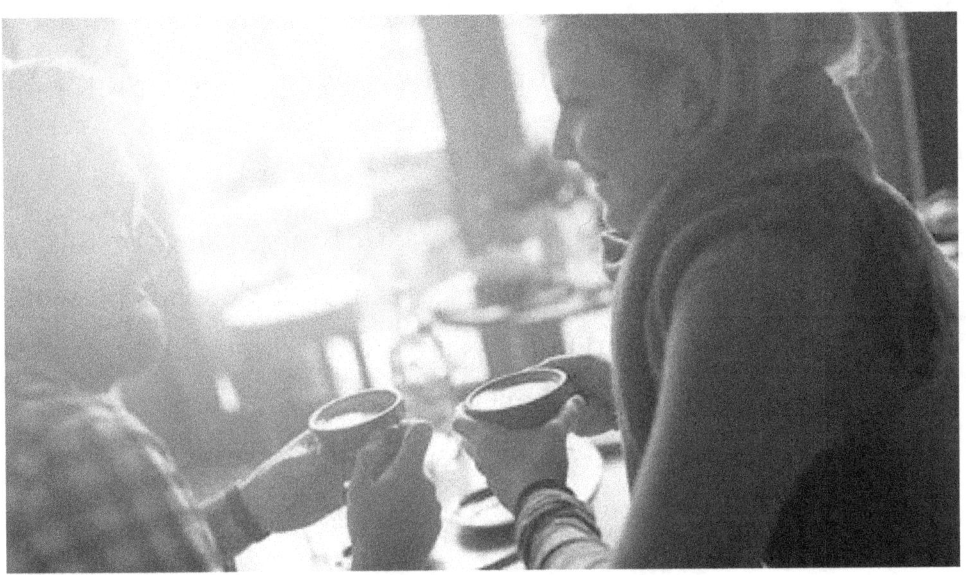

Let's suppose you've known your woman for a while, and you're excited to finally take her out. No matter where you meet your woman, when it is your first date, it is special. Whether you have met before or its your first blind date.

All you got to do is to start a conversation. The easiest and the best way to start the conversation with her on the first date is to find a natural compliment. Compliment her naturally. Tell her how pretty she looks. For example, you can start by saying, "Oh wow! You look gorgeous today."

Like the first time you met her, make small talk with her. And again, it could be anything like asking about the weather, work project, an event or just the latest news telecast.

When you left a good impression on her when you first approached her, this would be your first official date.

There will be chances of having a lot of more dates or this is going to be the last one with this woman. It all depends on what happens. There is a lot to impress a woman with in the first date. While most men work on their appearance, they forget to work on other things like what to talk about, how to react to different situations and what kinds of body language to use.

Women are very sensitive and if they find out that you just want to have sex with them then they will withdraw instantly. Men often make this mistake of showing how desperate they are. In other cases, some men like to brag about themselves. This is also a big turn off for women. Women don't like men who think too much of themselves.

If you want to tell a woman how generous you are then how it to her by your actions. Not by your words. Same goes for other things.

Your first date with a woman should be special for both of you. Choose a nice place where you two can have a good conversation. It shouldn't be too romantic and also not too casual. For example, some men make it way too fancy by choosing a place exclusively for themselves and decorating it with red balloons, etc. This would be too early for all that.

Also, the place shouldn't be informal like a bar or club. There would be too much background noise and you wouldn't be able to make an impact on her by engaging in a conversation. Something in between would be nice. A nice place for a dinner date would work perfectly fine.

The first date can be stressful. You should show confidence instead of telling her how nervous you are, and if you're not feeling confident, act confident anyway. Ask her about herself or talk about something of general interest, but don't focus on anything negative. Especially not about how anxious you are feeling.

However, if you are trying really hard to show you are relaxed and carefree, you might seem like you don't care, and she'll wonder why she's spending time with you.

This could be asking too much from a man, but try to find that balance. Show confidence, but make it clear that you're interested in her and have invested in winning her.

The way you start a conversation is very important. Ask her questions, and listen to her. Don't use your questions as an opportunity to launch into your own stories. And never try to dominate the conversation. Let it happen naturally, and if she's a good match for you, you'll enjoy the experience.

In the initial stages of dating, it is better to let her know that you're thinking about her and are interested in how her day was. Once you are done dating her, text her and share how much fun you had and that you're looking forward to seeing her again.

Sometimes, men play hard-to-get for the fear that they might seem too forward. But don't do that as it looks like you don't care. Whatever you do, don't be rude to women or ignore them to try to get a reaction. This way you would seem like a bad person. And this kind of behavior is ineffective and offensive. In such a case, she will not prolong the relationship with you.

Things to talk about

The most important thing you need to do is to make her feel attracted and respected when you meet a woman for the first time. Men often think being nice and friendly would make things work and she will be interested. It's a good idea to be that way of course, but there's more to it than just that.

If they don't find you attractive, they won't be interested in you no matter what you do and this may be your last date. When you first meet a woman, your aim should be to make her feel attracted towards you as you interact with her.

If you fail to make her feel attracted, it won't matter what you talk about as she will not be interested in what you say and do other than to be polite and friendly with you for a while.

Here are some tips on sparking up the conservation:

Focus on common interests

If she is someone you found on an online dating site, then recall the common interests you both share and start a conversation on one of those interests. For example, if she wrote about a TV show or book that you have seen or read then start a conversation about it like, "You like that TV show? I love it too. That actor must get an award for his performance."

Be witty

Having a good time and enjoying your company is the best thing a woman can have on a date. Be witty and make her laugh with short stories or fun jokes. Make eye contact when she is laughing. Show her that all your attention is for her and you are really into her.

Women can read small details. She will be able to tell from the way you look at her that you are admiring her.

Admire her

Tell her that she looks beautiful. Tell her that the color she is wearing suits her or the way she smiles is so adorable. In the middle of the conversation, make eye contact with her and keep looking at her. When she asks you, what are you looking at, tell her she looks so beautiful you can't concentrate on anything else.

Women love attention and compliments. This will make her develop more interest in you.

Moreover, women enjoy being acknowledged and knowing that you like the way they look, their personalities, their taste for colors, their shoes, their purses, their dogs and everything about themselves and the choices they make. So, you should keep the conversation about her.

A woman will not wish to hang out with you for long if your conversations are complicated and do not connect her with the topic you are talking about. You might have a good knowledge about something, but if it's not her field of interest, you would be making it inconvenient and boring for her. It is ideal to ask for the things she is interested in before you come to the dating place.

Be honest. Instead of using manipulating statements or viewpoints, talk with her in a way that shows that you really trust her. This way she will find it relaxing and will reciprocate your trust.

How to create a good impression?

On your first date with that special woman, you will want to make a good impression on her. You could do that by the following gestures:

Select a right place for your first official date

The place you choose for your first date sets the mood for your woman. Unless you already know what type of activities she likes, it is best to pick a neutral, low-pressure place where you can focus on getting to know each other and figuring out how well you both connect.

For example, a lovely restaurant that has private rooms with nobody around could put you and her together with some soft music. Because it's more comfortable for a socially extroverted girl to sit in a private room on the first date as both you and her have something to talk about that both of you don't want the others to hear it rather than a shy introverted girl who doesn't want to sit in a noisy bar that can overwhelm her.

The last thing you want to do is go to a nice restaurant and discover before your food even has arrived that you two don't get along and it's not going to work. In this scenario, you're stuck for the rest of the meal with each other.

Give attention to your body language

The way you present yourself verbally and nonverbally creates an impact on the woman you are dating. Your body language and facial expressions are the loudest when you are communicating.

Sometimes, it may be out of your control to be aware of your body language and still act naturally, but all it takes is identifying the negative body language and altering it a little. For example:

Don't fold your arms when the woman you are dating is telling you something. Instead, tilt your head towards her. Lean in. These are nonverbal indicators which will show her that you like what she is saying and want to hear more.

Moreover, if you want to know if your woman is interested in what you're talking about, look for similar body language indicators. You may want to change the subject if your woman crosses her arms or her feet are facing away from you.

Body language tells you a lot about a person. Just telling someone verbally that you are interested is not enough. You have to make sure your body is saying it too for a woman to accept it. In order to send a positive vibe to the woman you are dating, let your body do the talking for you.

There are three body language signs:

Mirroring

When you silently copy the behaviors of the person you are with it is known as mirroring. For example, if they smile, you smile back. It is observed that the more a person is attracted to people, the more he mimics their behavior. If you struggle to express your feelings on a date, mirroring the woman's behavior is a great way to subconsciously show them you are interested.

Facing

When you face your entire body from head to toe towards the woman you are dating, it is known as fronting. Usually men subconsciously point their toes in the direction they want to go. So, if your woman stays engaged and points towards you, it is a great sign, as it indicates they are interested in you. Whereas if their toes are pointed at the exit, they might not be having a good time.

Tilting

Wherever you are, if the woman you are with leans towards you, it is a clear sign that she is attracted to you and wants to be closer to you. Whereas, if she sits far back in her chair or take a step back from you, it shows her discomfort with the environment or conversation.

Be interested

In order to be interesting, you have to be interested. Men usually enjoy talking about themselves. Ask the woman you are with about her and show that you are interested in her. This would make you more interesting. Being aloof only looks good on a magazine cover, but it is no fun for anyone in real life.

You should show interest in the topics that come up. Show some curiosity as it is exciting. Someone who is curious shows that he is intelligent. So, if your woman brings up something you know nothing about, rather than thinking you have nothing in common, ask for more information. Women are happy when they talk about topics they like and they will notice that you are not a dumb person. Most of us won't realize it, but it is a very important trait.

Fuel Desire

You can fuel desire. Desire is not only about how you look, but also about what you wear. Desire comes from you.

If you are a man who wants to be desired, you must feel the desire. And if you want to feel desire, you have to feel secure about yourself.

Men are open to desire when they feel confident, radiant and free. These qualities enable men to feel more secure in themselves and thus open the door for longing to come in.

This may require some work on yourself. Developing confidence may not be as easy as throwing on a great outfit or getting your hair done. However, it doesn't mean that you have to hide out until you're fully confident.

You may have one thing that, when you would do it, you would feel totally in your element. For some, it's dancing. A person who loves dancing may feel more confident and alive while dancing. It may work like magic for them. Even when they don't feel good about their physical appearance, getting out on the dance floor can wash all the negative feelings away. You can gently lead her to the dance floor, choose the point that is far from the center if she isn't confident enough, hold her hands, help her to slowly swing her body with simple footsteps to get her warmed up.

Likewise, think about what makes you feel in your element. If it's something two people can partake then that's a great dating suggestion. This would bring all kinds of positive vibes to your woman. You will feel better about yourself and the woman you are with will feel that confidence radiating from you.

Listen to her

Women love to be heard and be given attention. You can show her you are actually interested in what she is talking about with a smile and some facial expressions or gestures. It is important to make her feel that you are the luckiest guy on Earth to get such an opportunity to hear her out. Simply do this by making your face look surprised with a slight smile and eyes looking straight into her eyes. Keep it simple and light, don't overdo it.

Don't interrupt her while she is talking. Ask her questions about herself and ask for some opinions like where could you get the best coffee in the town or which shopping mall is her favorite. Women like it when men value their opinions.

Be a gentleman

You may find it to be old fashioned to behave like a gentleman, but this is what all women want from a man. A woman wants you to hold the door for her to enter a restaurant, help her with her coat, and pull out a chair for her.

A lot of men don't have these etiquettes in the modern society, so if you develop a habit of doing these gestures, women will fall for you instantly. These gestures show an appreciation for the delicate beauty of a woman.

Be punctual

Make sure you are not late on your first date because being late will leave a bad impression on her. She might think that you're not sincere about your efforts to be in a relationship with her.

Make her feel secure and comfortable

Your woman would want you to make her safety and comfort be your priorities. In order to assure her that she is safe and secure with you, make sure you give importance to her preferences, too.

Table manners

The right table manners leave a good impression on women. Give her a nice memory to look back on by presenting good table etiquettes. Don't pretend to be sophisticated. You can just keep your table manners in check by letting your woman order first. Don't talk with a mouth that is full of food. Don't look at your dish all the time, after each bite, look around or at her.

<u>Final things to do to make sure to have a next dates or go to the next level of a relationship</u>

First dates can be exciting or they may just be a big disappointment. Your first date can either be a success or you may have ended up making it a failure.

How can you know whether your first date was a success or not and whether you can take your relationship to the next level or not? Here are some advice and indications that you may have more dates and take your relationship to the next level:

Plan ahead for the date

It's your job to do some planning. Nothing's worse than getting in a man's car and hearing, "So, do you want to eat somewhere, or…".

Plan out each part of the evening. You don't have to go over the top on a first date, as that's actually a really bad move, but make sure you know where you're headed. Otherwise, things are going to get really awkward, really quickly. If you're having trouble thinking of ideas, try listening and focusing on what she's actually interested in. For instance, be thoughtful and suggest a restaurant based on previous conversations. This shows that you are a good listener.

You could be yourself

If you were able to be completely yourself on a first date, that means it was a really successful date. There is no way that this wouldn't result in a second date and then a third and then in a long-lasting relationship.

Men always hope to find themselves on a date where they don't have to hold back or hide anything. This isn't always as easy as it might seem because some women just don't seem to get you or understand you. So, if you could be yourself on the first date and you were able to show your true and real personality, then it's a success. But don't be too relaxed by showing off everything that you know are your bad habits or things that need being improved on like nail biting, arms folding, etc.

You laughed

If you laughed on a first date, that means it was a really, really good evening. And you probably can't wait to see this amazing woman again and laugh even more. Women also seek laughter and excitement in a relationship and if you are able to make her laugh, then there are chances she would seek a relationship with you. Don't laugh so loud. That could attract the other table's attention and embarrass her.

Chemistry

The chemistry of the brain plays an important role in why we feel a certain way about other people. A lot of dopamine is involved, when we feel good about someone. When a woman or man experiences any kind of pleasure including love, a chemical named dopamine is released by the brain.

Dopamine also increases the amount of testosterone the body produces. For example, when people sweat around someone they love, the reason behind it is the increased testosterone levels. This is also why people have a higher sex drive when their love has just begun. If you feel a bond with her which couldn't be defined, there are chances that she also feels the same way. This could be an indication that this relation can be prolonged and you could take it to the next level.

You couldn't keep track of time

If you spend time with someone and feel like zero time has passed the entire evening when it had really been about four to five hours, then there is pretty much a good chance that this relationship will last a long time. The same applies if you have lost track of time during your first date because you are having such a great conversation and good company. This is first date perfection and it is a dream for many out there.

Be flexible about paying

Men often insist on paying, but some women aren't into that. That's why don't make it a big deal. If you're sneaking over to grab the check from the waiter or making a big show out of pulling out your credit card, you are making a bad impression.

Instead, if she insists on going Dutch, go along with it. If she expects you to pay, go along with it. If you offer to pay and she refuses to let you, go along with it. It's really not very complicated.

On the way home

On the way you take her home, you can care for her by asking questions like: "Are you cold? If you're cold, please take my jacket," then, you can offer her your jacket. You can also ask more about her things such as her family to know more about her. Finally, when you get to the destination, after saying goodbye to her, don't forget to thank her for a wonderful night then kiss her and say: "What a lovely evening with such an adorable lady" with a thankful face.

Things to avoid and pay attention to

Here are few things you should absolutely avoid on your first date:

Never mention your ex.

Don't bring up your ex-girlfriends, and don't ask her about her ex-boyfriends. You might think that you're simply looking for common ground, but it comes off as a little bit strange. The biggest turnoff for a woman is mentioning your ex on a date. This may seem like a sign that you have not gotten completely over your ex and your current date is merely a rebound.

This may make a woman think about whether you are ready for someone new or not. Besides, if you talk about what you don't like about your ex and you share them with her, then there is a high chance that she will judge you a bad guy. To be honest, it is extremely unsettling, and it doesn't do much in the long run.

Do not drink too much.

Drinking should really be kept to a minimum and no more than two alcoholic beverages preferably. Excessive drinking could lead to nightmarish situations where you make decisions you normally wouldn't. A first date may turn into a one-night stand if you are drunk. The goal is to engage with the person by listening and speaking, and that's really hard to do if you are drunk.

Avoid talking about marriage and kids.

Never make a mistake of talking about marriage and kids on the first date. Don't ask about whether she's planning to have kids, whether she's picked out her wedding dress yet or where she wants to take the wedding photos. Leave it for the other dates. Don't rush things. Wait for the right time. Otherwise you will scare her away and make her think you are desperate and needy.

Do not keep bragging about yourself.

Many men try to brag about their professional skills in front of women. They think they are doing a great job but in reality, they are not. Imagine a man going on for four hours about the intricacies of Excel. It doesn't sound impressive, does it? When you speak about yourself always keep a balance.

Also ask questions about the other person. If you brag too much about yourself, she may think you are self-obsessed. While men are trying to make a good impression, they start talking about their career. However, instead of speaking about yourself, you should place the attention on the woman and keep her engaged by asking questions and having her speak about herself.

A woman loves to talk about herself. You will make a much better impression while learning some valuable info about your potential partner-to-be, if you don't dominate the conversation.

Don't use your phone while she is talking

Using your phone while on your first date may seem rude. The woman you are with may think you are not interested in her. It is probably a good idea to turn off your phone until the date is over.

Don't ask her to come to your place or go to hers

Take things slow. A first date is just to get to know each other. Don't rush into having sex. Don't make the blunder of asking her to come over or inviting yourself to her place.

Don't try to be someone you are not.

Don't try to act and pretend to be someone else. This will not be helpful in the long run. However, you can copy their words, life quotes or any other things you can easily say and follow.

Avoid talking about things that can lead to controversies.

While it's important for many people to know where their date stands on finances, religion, the future, or politics, but don't bring them up on the first date. It can lead to arguments and uncomfortable moments if the two of you don't exactly stand on the same ground.

Don't rush things up

You might think that this is going somewhere serious, and if it is, that's great. But don't try to mess up all of your ideal relationship attributes over a single cup of coffee. Just take a step back and enjoy the evening. In the initial dates, you should be trying to get to know each other on a very basic level. Don't get impatient and start pressing for personal details or relationship histories.

Chapter 4: Making love to her

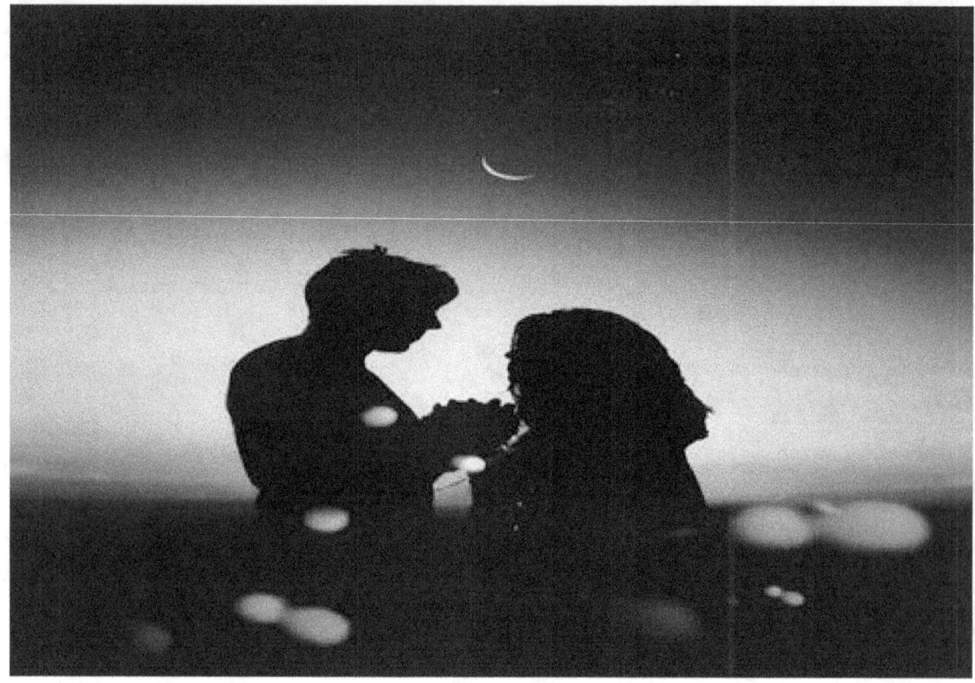

Women find sex to be the deepest form of love and connection, and many women are very sexually oriented while the others aren't. Women experience and express sexuality very differently from men.

Men often get disappointed that a woman doesn't crave sex as much as he does. This is because a woman's body is very different in terms of hormones. The male hormonal drive can be described as a loud yell, whereas a woman's is a whisper.

For a woman, what matters is how a man treats her and how he makes love to her. Therefore, a woman's appetite for sex is high when she is falling in love or is in infatuation period.

If a woman is ready to make love to you it means she has fallen for you and wants your love and affection. This can be the time when you could make her overwhelmed by your gestures. The way you make love to her will always be remembered by her. So, make sure you create a good impression on her.

There is a huge difference between having sex and making love like a man, and you have to understand this. Men can satisfy their sexual urges in a few minutes through straight intercourse. But love making is something more ornate. It will end later, but would start before the intercourse.

Women want their partners to make love to them. Making love to her will include everything from how you lead up to the moment to how much you focus on the foreplay to what you actually do while you are in the act and to how you end it responsibly.

The art of making love is not restricted to having sex. Foreplay is an important part of it and it can be more pleasurable than the actual act itself, especially for women. It is a way of making your woman ready for what is to come, and to build upon the anticipation. It is also a way for her body to prepare itself and start the natural process of lubricating, which will make sex more pleasurable and less painful.

Physical connect is not the only important thing in love making. You may have some amazing times in bed, but if you want to take it beyond that, the secret could be in connecting emotionally with her in bed.

Before the main event

If you and her can have some time before the main event at night, it is great. This is a good chance of warming her up. Women always desire love and care from the men they are about to engage. You can be tender by giving her some sexy words. For example, a scenario where you are sitting next to her in a park, you can lean towards her, then turn and kiss her saying, "I am sitting next to a super adorable lady." Later, you and her stand up and walk and then you can softly kiss her and say, "I love your scent." There is a high chance she will be pleased and ready for the next stage.

The truth about women is that they would love you more, and enjoy more in bed if you set up the mood for her. Depending on what she likes and how she likes to be pleased, create the perfect ambience for her.

Many couples want to take a bath before sex to warm up. If you and your woman enjoy this kind of warming up, you can consider filling up the bathtub and add some sensuous bath salts and a few rose petals in the water. Be sure that the water is relaxing and warm and help your woman step in the tub with you. Sit down with her and make eye contact. Tell her she is beautiful. Kiss her.

Women react to their surroundings differently than men. When it comes to making love, men react and behave differently than women. All a man can think about is sex. Whereas a woman wants intimacy before sex.

There are certain things which contribute to a woman's intimacy. These things include the decoration of the room. If you really want this to be memorable for your woman than decorate your room with scented candles and light them before you make love to her.

Dim the lights and light up a few scented candles around the house. Women love candles. Scented candles create an environment which arouses them. Use vanilla scented candles to really create an impact.

Add some slow and relaxing background music. And you will be surprised to see how she reacts to all this. If you want something new and more engaging, you can try some love making music on YouTube. If there is any music you don't know, use Shazam and make sure to have your phone near you so you won't miss the music. Some love dramas of the 80s and 90s have the most romantic music that you can look for and play them for your bedtime.

<u>Your words</u>

Your words matter the most to a woman, even when you are making love to them. Women love compliments. Tell her how attractive she looks. Flatter her by calling her beautiful. Tell her how nice she smells.

This would make her feel good and confident and would make her more aroused. She would respond more openly as this would boost her sexual confidence.

Communicate to her how great she is and how she makes you feel. The more you use words while making love to her, the more aroused she will get. Again, watch the love dramas of 80s and 90s, and you can find the best romantic quotes spoken by the male actors. So, spend your time watching them, noting down the quotes you like best and apply them for your bedtime. Pay attention to your tone and attitude when you say them. It must come from your true feelings. It is good that you can imagine the scenarios and practice them by thinking about them in your head, then act them out prior to the show time.

Your actions

Making love is the ultimate expression of the attraction felt between a man and a woman. It is the conclusion of an intricate relation that develops between a man and woman, starting with a simple look and evolving into a conversation, a touch, a kiss and finally into the shared expression of making love to each other.

It is a beautiful thing and is something that a man should really take care of when he is with a woman, which is what to say when in bed with a woman is so important.

Your relationship is defined when you're in bed with a woman. What you say to her really outlines your relationship. You can make her feel completely turned off or even hurt her emotionally. However, what is most important is your attitude.

A woman wants to see that you're relaxed, confident and totally attracted to her. What she sees, she will enjoy it more.

Confidence and attitude is what makes you good in bed. The less worried, hesitant and tense you are, the happier she will be and the more she will enjoy the sex and her time with you in the bedroom.

Fidget with her clothes

Some men have a habit of ripping off the clothes of a woman when they take her to bed. If you are one of those men who feel this is the best way to please your woman, think again because you might be wrong. There is a lot that you could do with the clothes of your woman before you take them off.

Instead of just removing all of the clothes at once or forcing her out of her clothes, turn this act into an act of sensual pleasure for her.

Take off her clothes slowly, making it enticing for her. Build up her mood. Give her a glimpse of what is yet to come. Move your fingers slowly by brushing her skin, and your lips should give her those pecks around the intimates, as she expects more of such acts while having sex.

Whatever she is wearing play along with it by taking out some of her clothes and leaving some on. For instance, if she is wearing a shirt and a bra underneath, slowly take her shirt off.

Use your teeth to open the buttons, move your fingers in a circle around her nipples, use your lips to play with her nipples, then lick, suck and give her little slight bites around her nipples and her stomach as you open her shirt. But don't hurt her with your bites. It's better to know her preference before you carry out the bites. Slowly massage her nipples and turn her on.

Once she has been turned on, you can remove the bra completely. Take her out of her lower dress and leave the panties on. You can slowly move your tongue over the panties, then her thigh till you can hear her moaning and writhing with pleasure.

Foreplay with her

Once she is wet move towards more foreplay. The word foreplay is strongly involved with pleasing a woman. Women like to enjoy the time they are in bed with a man, whereas men just like to do the act and get done with it.

Foreplay not only helps to set the mood, but it also prepares her body for sex. It makes her lubricate by making her wet. This results in feeling less pain during the intercourse. It also becomes more pleasurable for her when you finally do it.

Foreplay does not involve fingering her too tightly as that causes pain for her. Instead, you can gently rub her vagina to turn her on. Keep doing it softly.

You can also give her a sensuous massage, tease her by stroking her breasts with fingers, massage her nipples, then move your hands along her abdomen, hips and thighs while kissing those parts along the way. You can also touch her on her intimate parts down there in between the massage to help her get wet and get ready for the intercourse.

Don't hold your feelings and emotions back. Just groan while you are caressing her body. Say out loud any words, phrases and sentences reflecting your emotion with an emotional voice. For example, "Aargh, she is killing me!", "Oh dear! it's so good.", "Oh God, an angel is with me right here!" with a graceful gentle slow tone just a simple "aargh" while your lips are caressing her neck works very well.

Don't use bad language during this like the "F" word or other vulgar terms for sex. That is going to ruin the pleasant and loving mood you are trying to set.

When you go together with her through the stream of emotion, she will feel secure and trust you more. No ladies could resist when a man shows off all of his true feelings and love he wants to give to her.

Tease her into sex

Instead of rushing into sex right away, tease her into the act so that she enjoys it.

Make sure you do not leave any gap between foreplay and when you start having sex.

Once you start having sex, do not get rough and dirty immediately. Also, don't finish up the act quickly. Instead, keep it slow and prolong it.

A woman is almost at a point where she is ready to climax after oral sex, so you can start having sex then, but be slow. One method I suggest here is that each time of putting your penis into her vagina you don't need to put it in totally, maybe just half of it. Then the next time can be full penetration. Then you can make it in rhythm of half-full-half-full. You can choose any rhythm you like such as half-half-full or full-full-half. Stop once she gets in the mood, and then start again. Until she goes crazy and asks you to continue, then keep going on.

Please her in bed

Many women like when their men dominate them in bed, and it is a great way to turn her on.

Make sure that you keep her pleasures in mind and yet show her that you are with her. Hold her firmly in your arms and turn her around so as to play with any parts of her body. Be firm and strong, but do not hurt her in any way.

While you take control, talk to her and give her instructions about what she should and she should not do. For example, you can keep telling her to moan louder as you can see her reaching her climax, but tell her that she shouldn't hold your hands or use her hands when you want that. If one of her body parts is pressing against some of yours and causing pain, you can tell her about that. It's reasonable as each of you should be comfortable and happy while making love.

Notice how she laughs or smiles at something you say. Hold her gaze. Lean in a bit more. Touch her cheek. Tell her she's beautiful. Kiss her softly, on her lips. Don't make it hard. Keep it soft. Linger. Pull away a little. Let her see you. Let her lean in. Kiss her again. Let your lips linger. Take the lead and let her follow.

Pull her close; hold her by the waist. Don't force the touch; let it come naturally. Let her come closer. Notice her body language. Notice how she moves. Hold her in your arms gently. Trail a finger down her back. Make your skin the fabric of her dress. Run your fingers through her hair. Trail a finger along her jawline; hold her chin up to yours.

On the contrary, many women want to have control over their men. If she wants to be the leader of the game, just let her be. While being controlled by her, don't forget to do what she wants, caress her body while she is playing with your body and groan at each time she touches you. No matter how dominating your daily image is, in this case you can try being coy. It is very interesting and she will admire and love you even more as you let her control you. This is indeed a great way to show respect for her.

You can be flexible. In order to bring the new taste for your love, you can have intercourse in places other than the bedroom such as the kitchen, the garden or even in a remote forest or a secluded night coast on the weekends. Try new positions other than the traditional missionary like doggy, woman on top, etc. and find new ways to play with her body, for example, apply honey on her nipples then slowly consume it with your tongue or play with her nipples with ice.

Endgame

Stay with her after the intercourse has ended. Many women enjoy the moments with men after sex. Because while love is the sentence, sex is the full-on full stop. If you can fulfill the foreplay and the intercourse, it is great.

In both cases whether you can fulfill the intercourse or not, you should stay with her and fulfill the endgame responsibly. You can ask questions like "Are you still on it (her orgasm)?". In most of the cases, a woman's orgasm is longer than that of a man and she can have multiple orgasms besides the intercourse orgasm. Therefore, asking so shows her a huge respect for her feelings.

If she answers yes, then you may want to give an extra game by rubbing her vagina or carrying out another extra oral sex. You can ask her to lie on your body with her front body facing against the ceiling. Now you can do the rubbing with one hand. The other hand can caress all over her body. Some of the most sensitive parts are the breast, abdomen, and inner thigh. Your lips and tongue can also be used to kiss and lick her cheek and neck.

One of the most useful tips you can apply is that and you only keep her panties to the thigh level. Because if you remove the panties completely it is like a car without its break. In this case, the panties serve as a break. It helps her to avoid reaching orgasm too fast, hence, lengthens the play. The more elastic and comfortable the panties are the better.

In order to speed up and reach orgasm faster, she can straighten her legs, point her toes and clench her thighs and anus. When she wants to slow down, she can just simply stop pointing her toes, stop clenching her thighs and ask you to stop rubbing her vagina for a couple of seconds. So the orgasm will be on its way to reset a little bit. Then you and her can continue. I found this a most effective way to lengthen the play.

You can consider doing this extra play before the intercourse or after the intercourse or both, it's just the matter of preference.

At the end of the endgame, don't just rush into your blanket and sleep. Put your arm around her body, caress her gently, kiss and show her that it is a grace to your life that you are with her tonight.

Cultivating your love

After the night, you and her may have a chance of being peaceful together. This is a good chance to cultivate your love. Reviewing some of the conversations that you have loved from her is one of the great ways, for example, the first time you asked her out and she said "wow." You can say "I still remember the first time I asked you out and you said "wow." The way you said it was adorable. Remember when you repeat the main word, in this case is the "wow," try to make it sound as emotional as possible.

Another thing you can review is one of your first times of doing something. For instance, one of the first time you and her ordered chevon for your dinner and her sign is Capricorn. Then you can make fun comments on this by saying "I can't believe that I've caught this adorable goat" with a kiss. Surely, she will smile and fall for you.

The last but not least, there is possibility that she will tell you about her affairs. Congratulation if she does this. This means she trusts you and you are her man now so she can share with you her stories comfortably. Pay attention to her and express sympathy as well as cheer her up.

If you can fulfill your cultivation, it shows that you a profound man she cannot resist. Your relationship is ready for the next level.

Dos and Don'ts

the dos of making love

The way you look at her

The way you look at her while making love can get a woman more intimate with you. She may get turned on by the way you look at her. Make eye contact with her while making love to her.

Find out her erogenous parts

Women are different from men in many aspects. Men may not realize what a woman likes or dislikes. She may not like you touching her in some parts of her body.

You need to find the erogenous zones of her body. As not all women are aroused by being touched in the same zones. For example, one woman may adore having her breasts and nipples played with while a different woman may prefer you pay more attention to her vaginal region. One place most women get pleasure from is the clitoris, which is a part of the body men sometimes ignore. If you learn how to make her clitoris feel good, then you are going to be aces in her mind.

Give importance to foreplay and endgame

Men forget that women don't like to be treated as objects of pleasure. Therefore, go slow, and take your time. Build the mood and caress her. Foreplay and endgame make a great difference to women. To make her fall in love with you don't rush things and end them responsibly.

Talk to her

Many relationships have ended just because the men were in a hurry to leave. Women like a little cuddle and some talk while they are making love.
Say some sweet things to them. Your words would add to their intimacy.

The don'ts of making love

Don't complain about her

Making love to each other brings a man and a woman close to each other more than any sort of conversation can ever bring.

When you make love, you connect with each other on deeper, more primal levels as well as make each other feel amazing physically and emotionally. Do not criticize her in the bedroom. Focus your attention and energy on the things you find sexy about her and comment on that.

Don't talk about your ex

Never make this mistake of mentioning your ex while making love to a woman. It will not only turn her off, but also it will drive her away.

Don't try to end it in a hurry

If you are in a hurry don't rush things for her as well. A woman's body acts differently than a man's body. Give her some of her own time. Rushing things will lead to making a bad impression on her.

End Note

Women are different from men in all aspects and that is why men find it difficult to reach out to them. This book provides a complete set of guidelines, telling its readers how to develop a graceful image of that women find you attractive and how to successfully date a woman and finally make love to her.

A lot of men are unsuccessful in relationships and find it difficult to find women who are right for them. The book will help these men get into relationships with women successfully.

All they have to do is to read this book carefully and pay attention to the little details a woman gives importance to. It is very simple. If you want to get a woman fall in love with you, then you must love yourself. You have to enjoy your life and be happy with who you are. Until and unless you do that, getting a woman to love you will be not be truly possible. Enjoy life on your own even when women aren't in your life. Pursue the career, activities, and hobbies you enjoy. Volunteer for a cause you believe in. Surround yourself with fun, positive people who support you.

Summary of the important points

I have summarized for you all the important points that can give you a quick reference.

Women choose to be comfortable based on what kind of person they are around. They don't open up in front of men who just pursue sex. For men, everything is very straight forward. You may see a beautiful woman and feel aroused. Sometimes, you may pursue sex, but may not want to have a relationship with her. For a serious relationship with a woman, you may want to feel cared for, admired and respected by her and she wants the same from her man.

For women, it's different. They experience sexuality differently than men. This is why it is a lot more complicated for men to understand what really makes a woman get attracted to a man. Women fall for men who make them feel a certain way.

In order to develop emotions in a woman's heart you need to first determine the quality of the relationship you have with her. There are a number of ways to attract women. The way you choose will determine the type of woman you will attract.

For instance, if you try to attract women by choosing to be cold, calculating and manipulative, then you will only end up attracting a woman who is cold, calculating and manipulative. Likewise, if you want a woman because you are needy and you idealize them, then you will attract someone who is insecure and needy themselves. The same applies when you pursue a relationship with a woman with a harsh and rude manner. You will only attract a woman who responds to such emotions.

Women pay attention to little details. Your dressing style is one of them. You may not pay attention to what you are wearing. Men often have limited clothes and repeat the same shirts consecutively. This is because men do not find anything wrong with that. However, women are not like this. They will know exactly when you wore a particular shirt the last time.

The point is women notice your dressing style and in order to attract women you need to work on it. If you fail to style properly then you may fail to attract women. Your dress code should be on spot.

The correct gestures and the right body language are very important while attracting women. If you want to win over a woman you need to appear more masculine and confident. By using gestures and body language, you can silently communicate and make her fall for you.

Women like men who are confident. They would prefer talking to a person who believes in himself and knows his abilities. Show them you are confident by your body language. Stand straight with your shoulders up and hands out of your pocket. Make eye contact and keep eye contact when she is talking to you. Don't chase her.

Try to be a good listener. Show small gestures like opening the door for her, let her walk ahead of you, and offer your jacket if she is cold. In short be a gentleman.

Leaders are what women are looking for. If you have good leadership qualities and are always leading everyone whether it is a project, a sports game or anything you will find yourself to be known by women around you.

Becoming a leader takes ambition and body language. You can lead while interacting with a woman. However, there is a difference between leading and being bossy. Know the line between both. If you become dominating, then women will not be attracted to you and will be driven away from you.

You should show interest in the topics that come up. Show some curiosity as it is exciting. Someone who is curious shows that he is intelligent. So, if your woman brings up something you know nothing about, rather than thinking you have nothing in common, ask for more information. Women are happy when they talk about topics they like and they will notice that you are not a dumb person. Most of us wont realize it, but it is a very important trait.

On your first date, you must plan ahead for the date and be there on time. Try to be yourself, be flexible on paying and take her home. Once you reach the destination don't forget to say goodbye with a kiss and tell her that you've have a wonderful night with such an adorable lady.

Once you have taken your relationship to the next level it is time when you look forward to sex. Women find sex to be the deepest form of love and connection and many women are very sexually oriented. Women experience and express sexuality very differently from men.

Men often get disappointed that a woman doesn't crave sex as much as he does. This is because a woman's body is very different in terms of hormones. The male hormonal drive can be described as a loud yell, whereas a woman's is a whisper.

For a woman, what matters is how a man treats her and how he makes love to her. Therefore, a woman's appetite for sex is high when she is falling in love or is in an infatuation period.

If a woman is ready to make love to you, it means she has fallen for you and wants your love and affection. This can be the time when you could make her overwhelmed by your gestures. The way you make love to her will always be remembered by her. So, make sure you create a good impression on her.

Making love is the ultimate expression of the attraction felt between a man and a woman. It is the conclusion of an intricate relationship that develops between a man and woman, starting with a simple look and evolving into a conversation, a touch, a kiss and finally into the shared expression of making love to each other.

It is a beautiful thing and is something that a man should really take care of when he is with a woman, which is why what to say when in bed with a woman is so important.

Your words can cause her to feel an increased level of attraction, respect and love for you, or they can make her feel completely turned off or even hurt her emotionally. However, what is most important is your attitude.

A woman wants to see that you're relaxed, confident and totally attracted to her.

Finding the right woman and loving her may seem difficult, but it is not as hard as it sounds. Men just need to understand few things a woman likes, wants and hates is the key to her heart. Men may find it to be old fashioned to behave like a gentleman, but this is what all women want from a man. A woman wants you to hold the door for her to enter a restaurant, help her with her coat, and pull out a chair for her.

Very few men have these etiquettes in the modern society, so if you develop a habit of doing these gestures, women will fall for you instantly. These gestures show an appreciation for the delicate beauty of a woman.

Make sure you are not late on your first date because being late will leave a bad impression on her. She might think that you're not sincere about your efforts to be in a relationship with her.

Your woman would want you to make her safety and comfort be your priorities. In order to assure them that she is safe and secure with you make sure that you give importance to her preferences, too.

And finally, don't hold your emotions and feelings back. Merge yourself into the moments with her. No women can resist it when a man shows his true emotions, feelings and love for her.

All a woman needs are love and affection. If a man is successful in giving these two things to her. He will win her heart.

-- Hienel Farmrich

Bonus

I want to share with you some of my most romantic and loveliest experience I have had with my love. You can refer to these as to make your own moments of love. The message I want to convey is that sometimes the most romantic and loveliest things in love are just very simple. You just need to pay attention to and appreciate every single lovely moment you have.

On the motorcycle

It was a time she was driving her motorcycle and I was sitting behind her. It was one of the most interesting things I have done with my love. I sat behind her hugging her from behind. Then I kissed her cheek and pressed my cheek against hers. While pressing against her cheek, I closed my eyes. By that, I could totally merge myself into the moment with her. Another time when I was behind her, I stretched out my arms and said: "I am the happiest man in the world." In both times, my love was so excited as she could felt I had showed off all my true feelings.

Walking in the park

Another time I was walking in the park with her late at night and there weren't any other people. While walking, I played romantic pop music such as *My Heart Will Go On, Take My Breath Away, etc.*, while putting my arm around her. The atmosphere was much more romantic than the previous walks.

I did do that for my future wife

On one day, I helped her out with her documents. Then she said: "Thank you for spending time doing that for me. I have bothered you much" I replied: "I did do that for my future wife." I said the word "future wife" as emotional as possible while holding one of her hands. Then she hugged me from behind pressing her face against my back. I could feel she was very happy.

Have just woke up

One occasion when I visited her hometown, the bus reached the destination at 4 am and the trip was bumpy. So, I couldn't sleep on the bus. When we reached the house, we slept until 9 am. When I woke up, my face looked groggy and she found that was so adorable that she slightly slapped my face in the way of love then said, "oh dear look at your lovely face" with a cheek kiss. It was so adorable that I couldn't resist and had to hug her and kiss her back.

References

https://www.craigbeck.com/attracting-women-instantaneously/

https://www.fashionbeans.com/content/dating-mistakes-that-men-always-make/

https://www.luvze.com/impress-woman-work/

https://www.menshealth.com/sex-women/a25413723/how-to-ask-someone-out-date/

https://theartofcharm.com/art-of-dating/single-ladies/

https://visihow.com/Use_Scent_to_Attract_a_Woman

www.ingramcontent.com/pod-product-compliance
Lightning Source LLC
Chambersburg PA
CBHW050650250726
48662CB00002B/599